# Anti- Inflammatory Diet: The Long Term Benefits

## 30 Great Anti-Inflammatory Recipes

## By: Peyton Channing

# Publishers Notes

## Disclaimer

This publication is intended to provide helpful and informative material. It is not intended to diagnose, treat, cure, or prevent any health problem or condition, nor is intended to replace the advice of a physician. No action should be taken solely on the contents of this book. Always consult your physician or qualified health-care professional on any matters regarding your health and before adopting any suggestions in this book or drawing inferences from it.

The author and publisher specifically disclaim all responsibility for any liability, loss or risk, personal or otherwise, which is incurred as a consequence, directly or indirectly, from the use or application of any contents of this book.

Any and all product names referenced within this book are the trademarks of their respective owners. None of these owners have sponsored, authorized, endorsed, or approved this book.

Always read all information provided by the manufacturers' product labels before using their products. The author and publisher are not responsible for claims made by manufacturers.

**Paperback Edition**

Manufactured in the United States of America

# Dedication

This book is dedicated to my sister Alicia. She smiles through her pain and is never discouraged by her illness. She is s strong woman and I admire her for it.

# TABLE OF CONTENTS

**Publishers Notes** ........................................................................ 2

**Dedication** ................................................................................. 3

**Chapter 1-** The Anti-Inflammatory Diet ................................................ 5

**Chapter 2-** The Benefits of the Anti-Inflammatory Diet ................. 8

**Chapter 3-** Foods Allowed on the Anti-Inflammatory Diet..........12

**Chapter 4-** Foods Not Allowed on the Anti-Inflammatory Diet 17

**Chapter 5-** 10 Anti-Inflammatory Breakfast Recipes....................21

**Chapter 6-** 10 Anti Inflammatory Lunch Recipes ..........................28

**Chapter 7-** 10 Anti-Inflammatory Dinner Recipes ........................35

**About The Author** ....................................................................................43

# Chapter 1 - The Anti-Inflammatory Diet

Every so often a visit to the doctor will translate into advice to avoid certain foods. It might start with something as simple as reducing sodium intake due to hypertension, then go further on to sugar and carbohydrates for issues like diabetes. It may not be mandatory that we follow this advice; however, we all know that if we don't there will be consequences for us to deal with. In the same manner, an excessive amount of inflammation in the human body is counterproductive and can end up contributing to issues like cancer and obesity. Some foods that are loaded with saturated fat and sugar can act as triggers to this inflammation and drive the immune system in a direction that can make issues like arthritis a lot more unbearable and cause the body to slow down due to fatigue and could even be to the detriment of a few blood vessels.

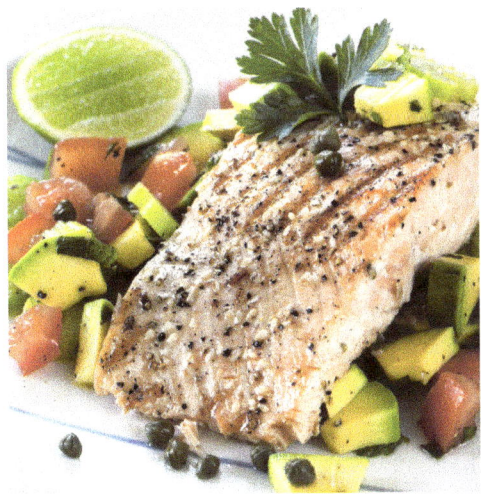

A successful anti-inflammatory diet is not for the purpose of losing weight, even though the word diet is included. Anti-inflammatory diets are designed to reduce the triggers that cause a flare up of inflammation and make for a healthier lifestyle and here are a few things to consider about such a diet. C-reactive protein has been known to trigger inflammation in the blood, avoiding excessive amounts of refined grains like pasta and rice and switching to whole grains instead is a start to breaking this cycle. Don't eat them all, but if you like nuts, specifically the ones that are high in fiber, such as walnuts and almonds you will be on the right track. For the most part, nuts are high in protein and antioxidants, with the latter being an excellent tool for the body to repair itself from some of the effects of inflammation, just stick to the good ones.

As children, we are told to eat our veggies and as adults we should be sticking to the same pattern, especially the dark and leafy kind. These veggies have phytochemicals, which are known to fight off diseases; they are also high in vitamin E, calcium and iron. Because of the fact that vitamin E has been known to fight off cytokines, which is a molecule that can cause inflammation, dark leafy greens are a must with this diet. Fish lovers should easily fit in with this diet especially if they prefer the fattier fish like sardines and tuna. Suggestions for an anti-inflammatory diet point to including fish at a minimum of twice a week, preferably more. When preparing the fish, stay away from frying the fish and avoid the salt, in preference to boiled or baked. Because fish has a high content of Omega-3, it is important enough to consider supplements if you don't like seafood.

All of your veggies do not have to be green and leafy, foods that are colorful are also important to include in your diet, especially since they are also known to be high in antioxidants. For the most part, bell peppers tend to fit the color requirement and the added advantage of being low in starch is definitely a plus. Some people prefer to get their colorful food from cayenne peppers and even chili, which include higher levels of capsaicin and is known to reduce inflammation. Another veggie that is not only colorful but tastes great is the tomato. Look for the juicy tomato; the redder the better and you will be adding a major weapon to your inflammation fighting tool chest in the form of lycopene. This is the kind of veggie that only increases in value after cooking it, however, either option will be acceptable.

There are several studies that point to soy as a great alternative to some of the foods that we eat, most people have already heard of soy burgers or soy milk. The greater health value derived from soy usually comes when there is not a lot of processing going on in exchange for the natural alternative. The benefits of soy to an anti-inflammatory diet can usually be seen in areas of the heart and bones. Maybe the Italians knew something that the rest of the world hadn't been made aware of until now and that is both garlic and onions provide the user with Ingredients that help boost the immune system. These two Ingredients also work similarly to pain medications that include NSAID to close avenues to increase the inflammation. Because of the fact that both onions and garlic can be effective in reducing inflammation and they improve the taste of every meal; they should be included in the anti-inflammatory diet.

There is a jingle that suggests that milk does a body good and while it may help with strong bones and teeth, the risk of casein and rheumatoid arthritis makes this food one to avoid. The good news is that if you are not affected by some of these triggers, a diet that includes low fat dairy products can reduce inflammation in the gut area. Another benefit of milk is the possibility of reducing the harmful effects of cancer. And finally, if you like cooking with oil, consider olive oil instead if only for the fact that it is healthier for the heart and better for reducing pain with inflammation. If olive oil is going to be on the menu, turn to the extra virgin option instead and take advantage of the fact that oleocanthal is included in this product.

# Chapter 2 - The Benefits of the Anti-Inflammatory Diet

You likely have heard of the anti-inflammatory diet before. With so many different diets out there and a new one touted almost every month or so, it can be difficult to know what benefits each diet has to offer and whether a diet plan is really right for you. The word "diet" has taken on a whole new meaning in the last ten years. The word "diet" no longer refers to simply a way to lose weight and improve health through weight loss. As I said in chapter 1, the word "diet" now often refers to a healthy eating lifestyle, one that can be maintained for life rather than something a person goes on and off repeatedly.

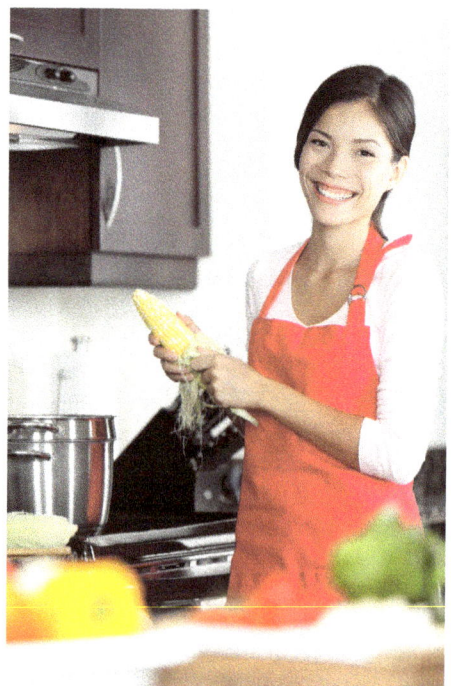

It can be complicated and time consuming to sort through the various diets out there and find a healthy eating plan that will work for you, but the anti-inflammatory diet can benefit absolutely everyone. This way of eating can help with many health issues that are extremely common and can improve conditions that we have come to consider as normal and acceptable in today's society. This diet can benefit multiple systems in the body including improving cardiac health, joint health and mental health. Here are some details on how you can improve your overall health through the anti-inflammatory diet.

The primary benefit of this eating style is that it can reduce your risk of getting heart disease. Heart disease is rampant with 1 in 4 deaths being attributed to this disease. Over 26 million people have been diagnosed with heart disease in the United States alone. Those are pretty staggering numbers. Heart disease does not discriminate and can affect anyone. Because this disease is so widespread, the possibility of reducing your risk of getting heart disease through a healthier eating plan is very encouraging and something we all should work towards.

Another benefit of this diet plan is the ability to lower your triglyceride levels naturally. Lipids are necessary, but when they become too high they can put a person at higher risk for developing heart disease. Many people struggle to keep their triglycerides at a healthy level and often prescription medication is needed to help control this. There are no symptoms that come with a high triglyceride level. Therefore, eating a healthy diet to help prevent elevated triglycerides and monitoring your lipid levels on a routine basis are great ways to try to prevent triglycerides from becoming too high and possibly leading to heart disease.

In addition, a person's blood pressure can be kept in check with the anti-inflammatory diet. We have all heard of high blood pressure as being a silent killer. Just as with high triglycerides, high blood pressure can also be present without any symptoms being shown. Due to the pressure that is applied to the arteries in a person with elevated blood pressure, the arteries can become weak which can ultimately result in death. Taking on a healthy eating lifestyle, such as the anti-inflammatory diet, can reduce your risk of developing high blood pressure, help to keep your blood pressure within a normal range, and result in maintaining healthy arteries.

A person with existing cardiac issues can also be rewarded by taking part in the anti-inflammatory diet. Because the diet helps control your blood pressure and triglycerides, and lowers the risk of heart disease, it in turn helps with any current cardiac problems a person may have. A healthy diet is a wonderful, natural way to try to keep your cardiac health stable.

In addition, this eating plan for life can give relief to stiff, aching, and painful joints. Anyone who suffers from arthritis can attest to the pain and discomfort that comes from even the most basic of daily activities such as bending, kneeling, sitting and walking. The capability to decrease the amount and severity of discomfort experienced on a day-to-day basis through choosing a healthy diet is a simple, practical way to live a little more pain free.

An anti-inflammatory diet can also help treat and prevent depression. Statistics show that 1 in 10 adults reports having depression at some point. Many of those have gone on to receive medical treatment through a variety of anti-depressant drugs, which need to be monitored closely. Because of the side effects associated with many anti-depressant medications, the option of possibly treating depression with diet, rather than drugs, may be a viable choice for some people.

Obviously, there are numerous benefits to your cardiac health with this eating lifestyle. While this set of benefits may not be the things you will see on a daily basis, the results will show through in your routine laboratory tests with lower triglyceride levels. In addition, each time your blood pressure is taken you may notice the benefit of your food choices; these work together to decrease your risk of heart disease resulting in an extended, improved life.

Unlike the cardiology benefits, a person with a diagnosis of arthritis will physically be able to notice the decrease in joint pain and stiffness typically associated with movements. Likewise, someone with a diagnosis of depression may notice improvement in their mood and affect, which can make all the difference in the world.

As you can see, the anti-inflammatory diet can improve your health in many ways. The option of being able to manage a variety of common health problems by simply choosing a healthier eating plan makes the anti-inflammatory diet a simple approach to healthier living. In the upcoming chapter you will learn more about the foods that can be consumed while on the anti-inflammatory diet.

# Chapter 3- Foods Allowed on the Anti-Inflammatory Diet

Inflammation and pain typically go hand in hand. When the fires of inflammation erupt all over a person's body, it can make one's life miserable, if not downright painful. It is not difficult for most people to recognize an achy muscle here or a sore inflamed joint there. Many of these aches and pains people get used to having. They expect that the pain will just always be there. Or they simply accept these regular painful sore spots as a state of normality for them--especially if the soreness appears in an area where an old injury once occurred. Others get pain that seems to move from place to place in their body, rather than sticking around in any particular spot.

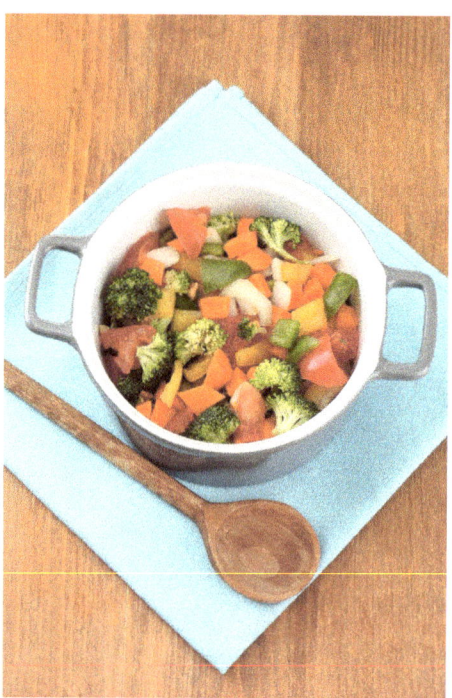

The more the person thinks about it, the more sore spots seem to appear. Many people would do anything just to feel pain-free again. When people are desperate for pain relief, they will try anything and pay any price for pills, creams, and even shots to alleviate the problem. The big pharmaceutical companies are certainly happy to flood the market with products which claim to be able to meet this unceasing demand. However, more often than not, the pain simply comes back. For the majority of people, eating anti-inflammatory foods would significantly help to put inflammation at bay. Like many other bodily responses, the inflammatory response in the human body can be significantly moderated by one's diet. In other words, it is possible to turn the inflammation response down significantly and live with reduced pain or in some cases totally pain free. But, which foods have the ability to tone down the body's inflammation response? Which foods can bring a person's sensation of pain back to a tolerable range?

*Foods Rich in Long Chain Omega-3 Fatty Acids*

Imagine a chain of atoms. Not just any atoms, but specifically carbon, oxygen, and hydrogen. Add a carboxyl group to the end of this chain, and what one gets is a fatty acid. Of course, there are many types of fatty acids. The number of carbon atoms in the chain plays a significant role in determining which type of fatty acid we are dealing with. The number of double bonds which reside in the molecule also helps to make this determination. The media has popularized Omega-3, omega-6, and omega-9 fatty acids in recent years. Come to find out, one of the most effective ways to combat inflammation is to up one's intake of Omega-3 fatty acids. Specifically, the Omega-3 fatty acid known as docosahexaenoic acid, which is often simply referred to as DHA in scientific literature. Deficiencies in this particular Omega-3 fatty acid have been associated with more than simply a rise in inflammation disease. Many other disorders, such as the rise in cardiovascular disease and neurological problems also result from a deficiency in

*Anti- Inflammatory Diet*

DHA. One can imagine then how critical it is to get a sufficient amount of DHA, which some scientists now argue, is an essential nutrient that all humans need.

Are plant derived Omega-3 fatty acids good enough? A plant derived short chain Omega-3 fatty acid, namely alpha-linolenic acid, often referred to as ALA, can be found in many plant based food sources, such as flax seed, wall nuts, and hemp seeds. Unfortunately, ALA needs to be converted to a longer chain Omega-3 fatty acid, such as DHA, before the body can truly gain any significant anti-inflammatory benefits. While it is certainly possible for the body to make this conversion, the amount of long chain Omega-3 DHA that is created by this process is too insignificant to produce any real therapeutic benefit. It is actually easier to get significant amounts of DHA from fish, fish oil, and krill oil, than from any plant source. Consequently, a diet rich in fish that contains a lot of Omega-3 fatty acids in the form of DHA is an essential foundation for reducing the inflammation and pain which many people suffer with every day.

*Probiotics and Inflammation*

Another anti-inflammatory substance, used in particular to combat the inflammation associated with Celiac disease, are probiotics. It is believed that probiotics can help reduce other forms of inflammation as well. When people think of taking probiotics, they either imagine popping a pill or eating yogurt as a source of dietary probiotics. But, what many people do not realize is that fermented foods, such as properly prepared sauerkraut and Kim chi also contain active probiotics. In modern times, we rely on cold storage to keep our vegetables fresh, so people today typically do not practice the art of making their own fermented foods as they did before modern refrigeration became popular for food storage. A lot of jar and can based fermented food storage processes, employed by food manufacturing companies involve heating, which destroys the beneficial probiotics in many of these fermented foods. If you can't find these products in a raw or unpasteurized state at the store, you can always learn to ferment these foods yourself. This is perhaps the best path to take to ensure the quality of the fermented food and that the probiotic content is still there when you are ready to eat it. This should help to ensure the maximum anti-inflammatory benefits possible. Plus, additional probiotics in one's diet can improve digestion and even help to take the edge off of inflammatory conditions like allergies and asthma.

<u>Foods Rich in Certain Antioxidants</u>

Antioxidants, often derived from fruits and vegetables, are organic compounds found in the foods people eat. When a person hears the word antioxidant, it is common to bring nutrients, such as vitamin A, C, and E or beta-carotene, to mind. These compounds are often thought of as being used to reduce the amount of free radicals causing cell damage in the human body. Yet, certain antioxidants, such as Alpha-Tocopherol, CoQ 9, and CoQ 10 have been shown experimentally to have an anti-inflammatory effect in mice, which is potentially good news for people who suffer with chronic inflammation. The implication is that eating foods or taking supplements rich in these antioxidants may help to prevent or lessen the severity of inflammation in humans as well. In particular, Alpha-Tocopherol, also known as vitamin E, can be found in foods like Avocados, egg yolks, Kiwi, red peppers, and spinach just to name a few dietary sources.

Of course, there are other foods, such as certain types of mushrooms, herbs, and such that are also said to have anti-inflammatory properties. Hence, if a person is getting a wide enough variety of these foods, they should begin to notice a

*Anti- Inflammatory Diet*

significant decrease in inflammation as well as pain. For many people it is not so much that they never get these nutrients in their diet. Rather, the problem tends to be that they do not get them in high enough of a quantity to make a difference. If a person suspects that this is the case, he/she can always search around for supplements that contain the active anti-inflammatory Ingredients: they need in a more concentrated form.

# Chapter 4- Foods Not Allowed on the Anti-Inflammatory Diet

In the previous chapter, you learnt about the foods that are allowed on the anti-inflammatory diet. Let's now take a look at the foods that are not allowed on the anti-inflammatory diet. There are many websites out there that promise rapid weight loss, with catchy names and high hopes of easy success. They also typically promise not only weight loss, but better health, increased energy, and an abundance of happiness when the weight is gone! But what it usually comes down to is this: eat whole grains, lean meats, more greens, and drink lots of water. This is also the basis for the anti-inflammatory diet, but this plan promotes more than just weight loss.

The anti-inflammatory diet, or rather, anti-inflammatory eating, is also based on the idea of eating healthy for life. The main point of the diet is that when the body is in a state of constant inflammation, it leads to various illnesses, but that this can be controlled by eating correctly. Better eating equals weight loss, which equals better health and less chance of developing a disease. Inflammation is not just a problem for those suffering from arthritis or sore muscles; it can also be a factor for strokes, heart attacks, and cardiac problems. As mentioned in chapter 2, supporters of the anti-inflammatory diet state that it can reduce the risk of heart disease, lower blood pressure and blood triglycerides, and relieve even the stiffest and sorest of arthritic joints.

Knowing what not to eat on the anti-inflammatory diet is just as important (if not more) as knowing what can be eaten. It's easy to make a list of all the items that can be bought at the grocery store to stay on a diet. Knowing what to avoid can be harder, especially when so many common household foods contain Ingredients that are not permitted on this healthy eating plan. It takes research and patience, but the rewards are worth it in the long run.

*Anti- Inflammatory Diet*

Refined and high glycemic carbohydrates are ones that can be rapidly broken down into simple sugars. When broken down, they enter the bloodstream quickly, causing blood insulin levels to spike. These carbohydrates can be very addictive, and unfortunately, they are everywhere. Carbs to avoid are:

- Table sugar
- Fruit juice
- Cookies
- Cakes
- Pies
- Chocolate
- Jelly
- Jams
- White bread
- White rice
- Soda
- Potato chips
- High fructose corn syrup
- Pastas made with white flour
- Apples
- Bananas
- Granola
- Dried fruits

Fruits and vegetables are generally a good addition to any diet, or healthy eating plan. But there are some that have a high glycemic index, and should be avoided on the anti-inflammatory diet. Apples and bananas were mentioned before, as these two also have a high sugar count. Other fruits and vegetables to avoid are:

- Cantaloupe
- Pineapple
- Watermelon
- Carrots
- Beets
- White potatoes
- Parsnips
- Peas
- Acorn squash
- Corn

Red meats are to be strictly avoided when on the anti-inflammatory diet. Red meat is the darker colored meats that come from cows, sheep, and horses. Studies of red meat have shown links to inflammation caused by arthritis, as well as cancer, so cutting them out in this diet is an important step. Avoid:

- Beef
- Pork
- Lamb
- Mutton

Processed foods are another area to avoid on the anti-inflammatory diet. This one is tricky, as these types of food are usually the convenience foods that are packaged to last longer and are typically loaded with artificial preservatives. They are usually very low in nutrients, and many are high in salt, neither of which is good for the body. Many also contain too many omega-6 fatty acids. Avoiding them on this diet is essential for success, so look out for:

| | |
|---|---|
| • Hot dogs | • Boxed dinner mixes |
| • Lunch meats | • Fast foods |
| • Granola bars | • Diet foods |
| • Breakfast cereals | • White bread |
| • Artificial sweeteners | • Vegetable oils |

This is just a small list of the processed foods that are popular today. The best way to determine whether a food is processed or not, is to examine the ingredient list. The longer it is, the more processed. You'll also want to be able to pronounce the items in the list, and know exactly what they are.

Saturated and trans fats must also be avoided in order to maintain the anti-inflammatory diet. Too much saturated fat can raise the cholesterol levels in your body, which then can lead to increased risk of stroke and heart disease. Saturated fats occur naturally in a lot of common foods. The AHA, or American Heart Association, recommends a daily limit of saturated fat to remain under 7% of all calories. Look to avoid:

- Butter
- Cheese
- Cream
- Whipped cream
- Poultry with skin
- Fatty beef
- Fried foods
- Eggs
- Bacon
- Palm and coconut oil
- Sardines
- Sausage
- Macadamia and brazil nuts

Know your spices. It's easy to grab the salt and pepper shaker to spice up a meal. But salt is a definite ingredient to avoid, as too much sodium can cause high blood pressure, edema, breathing problems, and more. Instead, stock up on natural inflammatory spices such as ginger and curry.

Inflammation plays much more of a harmful role than what was previously thought, according to the experts. Those who are heavier are at a higher risk of suffering from arthritis, which is one of the leading causes of inflammation. The anti-inflammatory diet is one that can be used to kill two birds with one stone; first, as a weight loss plan, and second, as a health plan. Talk to your doctor before starting any weight loss program, and be sure to stay under their care as you progress. With diligence, this diet can produce results not only aimed at weight loss, but at better health and well-being, as well.

# CHAPTER 5- 10 ANTI-INFLAMMATORY BREAKFAST RECIPES

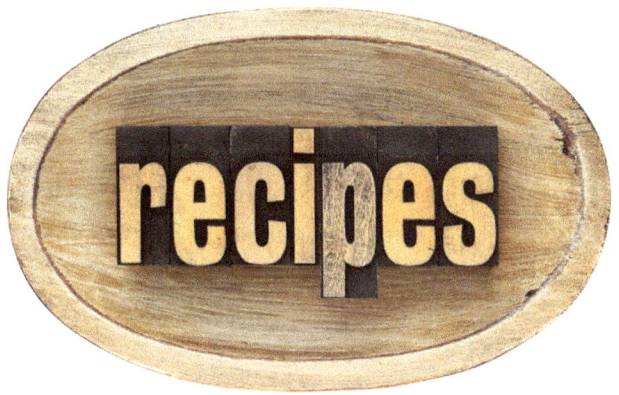

### *Egg In A Hole*

Ingredients:

- 1 egg
- 1 slice bread, whole grain
- Small amount of butter for frying

Instructions:

- In nonstick frying pan, melt butter over medium heat.
- Create a one-inch hole in the center of the bread and place it and the punched out hole of bread in pan. A cookie cutter or open end of a glass will create a uniform hole.
- Drop egg into the hole in the slice of bread and fry for 1 ½ minutes on each side.
- 4. May serve with ham or bacon on the side.

### *Breakfast Smoothie*

*Anti- Inflammatory Diet*
Ingredients:

- 1 banana
- 1 Cup orange juice
- 2 and 1/2 cups frozen berries
- 1/2 cup low-fat yogurt (plain)

Instructions:

- Transfer orange juice into blender. Add yogurt to orange juice in blender until the liquid level is at the one and a half cup line.
- Place in bananas with the yogurt and orange juice mixture. Puree slightly.
- Place in Strawberries until the liquid reaches the four and a half cup line on blender cup. Blend until smooth.

Add more strawberries if necessary to meet the four cup line on blender.

## **Breakfast Berry Crisp**

Ingredients:

- 1 Cup of blueberries
- 1 Cup of raspberries
- 2 cups of halved frozen or fresh strawberries
- 1/4 cup of corn starch
- 4 tsp. of sugar
- 1/2 tsp. salt
- 1/2 tsp. cinnamon
- 1 Cup rolled oats uncooked
- 1/2 cup packed dark brown sugar
- 1/3 cup flour whole wheat

- 1/2 cup walnuts or pecans
- 5 tbsp. butter

Instructions:

- Pre-heat oven to 350 degrees.
- In large bowl, place berries, oats, sugar and corn starch. Toss to coat. Add more sugar if tart berries are the prominent berries in the mix.
- Empty contents of the bowl into a baking dish.
- In same bowl, place oats, brown sugar, flour, salt, cinnamon, and pecans.
- Cut cold butter into the flour mixture until a course meal state. Incorporate by hand or with cutter.
- Sprinkle evenly over the top of the berry mixture without packing berries down.
- Place in 350-degree oven for 35 minutes. The top will brown and the berries will bubble up.

### ***Spinach Egg Bake***

Ingredients:

- 12 slices of cooked and crumbled slices of turkey bacon
- 2 packages spinach, frozen
- 8 oz. of parmesan cheese
- 12 eggs

Instructions:

- Preheat oven to 400 degrees.
- In large bowl, mix all Ingredients.
- Spray 9 x 12 baking pan with non-stick spray.
- Pour contents of bowl into pan.

- Bake for twenty-five to thirty minutes. After cooling, cut into serving size pieces.

### Pizza Omelet

Ingredients:

- 9 pepperoni slices
- 1/4 cup mushroom pieces
- 3 eggs, large
- 1/8 cup choice spaghetti sauce
- 2 oz. of mozzarella cheese
- 1 oz. of milk, 2%

Instructions:

- Whisk together milk and eggs. Season with salt and pepper.
- Pre-heat and grease a fry pan.
- Add egg mixture to hot pan.
- On 1/2 of the egg mixture, layer the mushrooms, cheese, and pepperoni slices.
- When the egg is done, fold plain side of egg on top of cheese side.
- After plating, spoon some spaghetti sauce over the top before serving.

### Soy Protein Pancakes

Ingredients:

- Water
- 1 tbsp. powder soy protein
- 1 egg or two egg whites
- 1/4 cup cottage cheese, fat-free

- 1/4 cup oatmeal
- Vanilla, maple extract, ground cinnamon (to taste)

Instructions:

- In blender, mix all Ingredients: until mixture reaches a batter consistency.
- Spray coating on frying pan.
- Pour batter into hot pan until edges are brown. Flip pancake over for additional browning.
- Top with fruit, applesauce, or sugar-free syrup.

### **Strawberry Yogurt Breakfast Split**

Ingredients:

- 1 tbsp. sliced almonds
- 1 Cup fresh or frozen strawberries
- 1 banana
- 1/2 cup plain or vanilla yogurt

Instructions:

- Cut banana in half and place in serving dish.
- Place dollops of yogurt along center of bananas. Sprinkle strawberries and almonds to the top of the center of the bowl.

### **Radish Hash Browns**

Ingredients:

- 1/4 of finely sliced medium onion
- Pepper and salt (to taste)

*Anti- Inflammatory Diet*

- 1/2 pound grated red radishes
- Paprika to taste (pinch or two)

Instructions:

- Spray oil into fry pan and heat up.
- Cook onions with a small amount of water until translucent.
- Add radishes to pan and continue to cook. The color of the radish will deepen and they will crisp when done.
- Serve as a side dish with other breakfast items.

### **_Creamy Salmon Spread_**

Ingredients:

- 3/4 tbsp. lemon juice
- 3 oz. of cream cheese, fat-free
- 1 tsp. Worcestershire
- 1 tsp. dried dill weed
- 2 oz. of pink salmon, chunck style skinless and boneless

Instructions:

- In a large bowl, mix all Ingredients: together.
- Place in refrigerator and let set overnight to marry the flavors.
- Offer as a spread on Melba toast or whole wheat bagels. Great for a quick breakfast on the go or even for a light lunch or afternoon snack.

### **_Granola Go Cup_**

Ingredients:

*Peyton Channing*
- 1/2 cup blueberries
- 1/2 cup raspberries
- 1/3 cup low fat granola
- 1 Cup non-fat vanilla yogurt

Instructions:

- In a large bowl, mix together fruit, yogurt, and granola into plastic cups. Place into the cup in this order: yogurt, fruit, and granola.
- Chill slightly. Can be eaten for a healthy breakfast or packed up and taken on the go.

# Chapter 6 - 10 Anti Inflammatory Lunch Recipes

### *Waldorf Salad*

Ingredients:

- 12 seedless purple grapes, halved lengthwise
- 1 apple, peeled and diced
- 1 cup coarsely chopped fennel bulb
- 1 tbsp. freshly snipped parsley
- 2 tsp. unsalted sunflower seeds (optional)
- 2 tsp. fat-free mayonnaise
- 1/4 tsp. dried dill weed
- Romaine lettuce

Instructions:

- In a medium bowl, combine grapes, apple, fennel, parsley, sunflower seeds (if using), mayonnaise and dill weed.
- Serve on beds of Romaine lettuce.

### *Sicilian Spinach Bread*

Ingredients:

- 1 tbsp. extra-virgin olive oil
- 10 oz. fresh spinach, trimmed and finely chopped
- 1 large French baguette
- 2 tbsp. light margarine
- 1/2 cup low-fat shredded mozzarella cheese

Instructions:

- Preheat oven to 375 degrees

- In a medium saucepan, heat oil over high heat.
- Sauté spinach, and salt to taste for 5 to 7 minutes, or until wilted. Remove from heat.
- Slice baguette in half lengthwise.
- Spread margarine and spinach mixture over each half. Sprinkle with cheese.
- Sandwich the two halves with topping pressed together and wrap in foil.
- Bake in preheated oven for 10 minutes.
- Spread the foil open and bake for 5 minutes longer, or until bread is hot.
- Cut into 2-inch thick slices.

## *Light Crab Chowder*

Ingredients:

- 3 large potatoes, peeled and chopped
- 2 carrots, peeled and finely sliced
- 1 stalk celery, finely sliced
- 2 cups vegetable stock
- 2 tbsp. snipped fresh parsley
- drained, canned crab meat
- 1/2 cup 1% milk or lactose-free 1% milk
- 1 tbsp. all-purpose flour

Instructions:

- Spray a medium saucepan with vegetable cooking spray and heat over high heat.
- Sauté potatoes, carrots and celery for 3 to 5 minutes, or until slightly softened.
- Add stock, parsley, and salt to taste.

*Anti- Inflammatory Diet*

- Reduce heat to medium-low and simmer, partially covered, for 35 minutes, until vegetables are tender.
- In a small bowl, whisk together crab meat, milk and flour until smooth.
- Gradually add to pot and simmer, stirring frequently to prevent clumps, for about 10 minutes, until thickened.

### **<u>Vegetable Spring Rolls</u>**

Ingredients:

- 6 mushrooms
- 1 red bell pepper, halved and seeds removed
- 2 cups baby bok choy, finely sliced
- 1/2 cup diced tofu
- 2 tbsp. reduced sodium soy sauce
- 8 large round rice paper wraps

Instructions:

- Grill mushrooms and red pepper for 6 to 8 minutes, or until mushrooms are tender and skin of pepper is blistered and brown.
- Let cool and slice mushrooms and pepper lengthwise.
- Spray a wok or skillet with vegetable cooking spray and heat over high heat.
- Stir-fry bok choy, tofu and soy sauce for 6 to 8 minutes or until vegetables are tender.
- Let cool slightly.
- Working with one rice paper, soak in warm water for 5 seconds. Gently remove and lay on a flat surface.

- Place 2 tbsp. vegetable mixture on the bottom edge of each wrap and fold left and right sides over filling, making a rectangle.
- Starting at bottom, roll up into cylinder to enclose filling.

## *Mango Chicken*

Ingredients:

- 2 boneless chicken breasts
- Pinch ground ginger
- 3 canned mango slices, cut into matchsticks
- 1/4 cup canned mango liquid
- snipped fresh cilantro

Instructions:

- Preheat oven to 375 degrees; 11 x 7 ungreased baking dish.
- Place chicken breasts in baking dish and sprinkle with ginger and salt to taste.
- Cover with mango slices, mango liquid and cilantro to taste.
- Bake in preheated oven for 30 to 40 minutes, or until chicken reaches an internal temperature of 170 degrees Fahrenheit and is no longer pink inside.

## *Baked Chicken Fingers*

Ingredients:

- 3 large boneless, skinless chicken breasts
- 1/4 cup liquid egg whites, lightly beaten
- 1/2 cup seasoned dry bread crumbs
- 1 tsp. olive oil (optional)

*Anti- Inflammatory Diet*

Instructions:

- Preheat oven to 375 degrees; baking sheet, lightly greased
- Slice chicken breasts in long slices, 1 inch thick.
- Dip each piece in egg white, turning to coat, then dredge in bread crumbs until evenly coated.
- Place on prepared baking sheet and drizzle with oil, if using.
- Discard any excess egg white and bread crumbs.
- Bake in preheated oven for 20 to 25 minutes, or until chicken is no longer pink inside and coating is crispy.

### ***Fishy Rice***

Ingredients:

- 1 large carrot, peeled and grated
- 1 1/2 cups coarsely chopped spinach
- 1 can flaked water-packed tuna, drained
- 3 cups chicken stock
- 1 tbsp. snipped fresh parsley
- 3/4 cup long-grain white rice

Instructions:

- Spray a large saucepan with vegetable cooking spray and heat over high heat.
- Sauté' carrots and spinach for 3 minutes, until slightly softened.
- Add tuna, stock, and parsley. Reduce heat to medium-low and simmer, partially uncovered, for 15 minutes.
- In a pot of boiling salted water, cook rice for 12 to 15 minutes, or until tender.

- Drain rice and combine with tuna mixture. Serve immediately.

### Moroccan-Style Carrot Salad

Ingredients:

- 1 1/2 cups grated peeled carrots
- 1/3 cup golden raisins
- 2 tbsp. extra-virgin olive oil
- 1 tsp. honey
- 1/2 tsp. ground cinnamon

Instructions:

- In a medium bowl combine carrots, raising, 1/4 cup water, oil, honey, cinnamon and salt to taste.
- Cover and refrigerate for 1 hour. Serve chilled.

### Spinach with Raisins

Ingredients:

- 1 tbsp. canola oil
- 6 cups hand-torn spinach
- 1/4 cup golden raisins
- 1/4 pine nuts (optional)

Instructions:

- In a large skillet, heat oil over medium-high heat. Sauté spinach for 5 minutes, or until wilted.
- Add raisins, pine nuts (if using) and salt to taste; cook for 5 minutes, until pine nuts are softened.

*Anti- Inflammatory Diet*

## **Baked Butternut Squash**

Ingredients:

- 1 large butternut squash
- 1 tsp. light margarine
- 1/2 tsp. lightly packed brown sugar
- ground nutmeg

Instructions:

- Preheat oven to 375 degrees; 13 x 9 baking dish
- Slice butternut squash in half lengthwise and scoop out seeds.
- Dab margarine in the hollowed-out section of each half.
- Place in baking dish and sprinkle with brown sugar and salt and nutmeg to taste.
- Cover and bake in preheated oven for 45 to 50 minutes, or until tender.

# Chapter 7- 10 Anti-Inflammatory Dinner Recipes

### *Beef and Barley Stir Fry - Serves 2*

Ingredients:

- 1/4 cup Barley - pearled
- 1 Tomato - sliced
- 2 tsp. Olive Oil
- 7 oz. Lean Ground beef
- 1 cup Mushrooms
- 2 cups frozen Green Beans
- 1/4 cup Kitchen Basics unsalted vegetable stock
- 1/2 tsp. low sodium Soy Sauce

Instructions:

- Cook Barley according to package Instructions.
- Slice tomato, set aside.
- In large skillet heat oil to medium-high.
- Add ground beef. Stir and cook until browned.
- Add onion, mushrooms and green beans. Cook until beans are crisp tender.
- Stir vegetable stock and Soy Sauce in cooked barley.
- Add to the meat and veggies Serve with sliced tomato on the side.

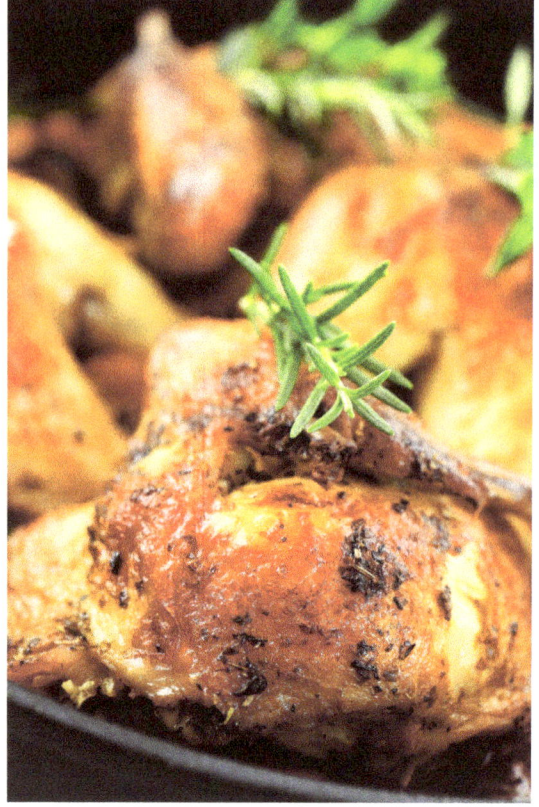

### *Almond Chicken - Serves 1*

Ingredients:

- 3 oz. boneless Chicken Breast – sliced
- 2 cups Broccoli flowerets – steamed
- 1 ½ tsp. Olive Oil
- 1 Green Bell Pepper and ¾ cup onion - both chopped
- 1 clove Garlic – minced
- 1 cup Cherry Tomatoes – halved

Instructions:

- Steam broccoli.
- In a sauté' pan heat Olive Oil.
- Add chicken, green pepper, red pepper, onion and garlic.
- Sauté' until vegetables are cooked al dente and chicken is cooked through.
- Add tomatoes and steamed broccoli. Top with almonds.

### **Baked Cod with Beans and Salad - Serves 1**

Ingredients:

- 2 tsp. Olive Oil - divided
- 1 tbsp. Old Fashioned Oatmeal
- 4 oz. Cod
- 2 slices Tomato
- 2 cups Green Beans
- 1 small Side Salad
- 1/2 cup Blueberries

Instructions:

- Preheat oven to 400 degrees Fahrenheit.
- Mix 1 tsp. Olive Oil and Oatmeal in a small dish.
- Add salt and pepper to taste.
- Place Cod in shallow baking dish and cover with oatmeal mixture.
- Place sliced tomatoes and onions atop Cod/Oatmeal. Bake until Cod flakes (about 15 to 20 minutes depending on thickness of Cod).
- Steam green beans. Top the salad with blueberries.
- Serve Cod with beans and Cottage cheese and Fruit Salad.

### **Cottage Cheese and Fruit Salad**

*Anti- Inflammatory Diet*
Ingredients:

- ¼ cup Low-fat Cottage Cheese
- 1/3 cup Mandarin Oranges canned in water
- 2 ½ tsp. slivered Almonds

Instructions:

- Mix Mandarin Orange sections in a bowl with the Low-fat Cottage Cheese.
- Top with slivered almonds.

## **_Weeknight Turkey Chili - Serves 6_**

Ingredients:

- Vegetable Cooking Spray
- 1 large Onion - chopped
- 1 tbsp. Garlic - minced
- 1 1/2 pounds Ground Turkey
- 2 cups water
- 1 28 oz. can crushed Tomatoes
- 1 16 once can Kidney Beans, drained and rinsed
- 2 tbsp. Chili Powder
- 2 tsp. Turmeric
- 1 tsp. each of Smoked Paprika, Dried Oregano, Ground Cumin, Hot Sauce

Instructions:

- In a large soup pot sprayed with cooking spray, cook onions until tender and starting to brown, about 5 minutes.
- Add garlic and cook 30 seconds.

- Add turkey and stir frequently until fully cooked, about 10 minutes.
- Add water and remaining Ingredients: and bring to boil.
- Reduce heat and simmer uncovered 30 to 45 minutes.

### *Kipper Salad - Serves 4*

Ingredients:

- 1/2 cup Reduced Fat Mayonnaise
- 1 small Onion and 1 Celery Stalk finely chopped
- 1 tbsp. chopped fresh Parsley
- 1 tsp. Lemon Juice
- 1 clove Garlic - minced
- 1/8 tsp. salt
- 1/8 tsp. ground Black Pepper
- 1 (6 oz. can) Kippers - drained

Instructions:

- In medium sized bowl, stir together first eight Ingredients.
- Add flaked Kippers and gently toss to combine.
- Refrigerate until ready to serve.

### *Eclectic Cabbage Soup – Serves 2*

Ingredients:

- 2 tsp. Olive Oil
- 6 oz. ground Turkey Breast
- ¾ cup Onions – diced
- 1/3 cup canned Garbanzo Beans – rinsed and drained
- 4 cups Cabbage – shredded

*Anti- Inflammatory Diet*

- 1 ½ cups Mushrooms – sliced
- 1 ½ cups Bell Peppers and 1 ¼ cups Tomatoes – diced
- 2 cloves Garlic – chopped
- 1/8 tsp. Caraway Seeds, 1/8 tsp. Tabasco Sauce and Salt and Pepper -all to taste
- 2 tsp. Virgin Olive Oil – Drizzle

Instructions:

- Brown meat and onions in Olive Oil.
- Add all other Ingredients: except Extra Virgin Olive Oil.
- Cover and let simmer until vegetables are cooked – at least half an hour, so that all flavors blend well. Drizzle with Olive Oil.

### ***Concetta's Leftover Quickie - Serves 2***

Ingredients:

- 2 tsp. Olive Oil
- 7 oz. extra firm Tofu - cut into cubes
- 1 cup Japanese Eggplant - thinly sliced
- 1 clove Garlic - diced
- 1 cup Zucchini - cooked, steamed
- 1 cup Cherry Tomatoes - halved
- 3 oz. Pork Loin - cooked
- 3/4 cup Garbanzo Beans (canned, rinsed drained)
- Salt and Pepper to taste
- 1/2 cup Grapes to share

Instructions:

- Heat oil to medium in large skillet.

- Add Tofu and eggplant. Sauté' until golden brown.
- Add Garlic and brown after a few minutes of cooking the Egg Plant mix.
- Add Garbanzo Beans, salt and pepper.
- Toss well together and serve luke warm.
- Share a few grapes.

### Chicken and Green Beans Italian Style - Serves 1

Ingredients:

- 2 tsp. Olive Oil
- 3/4 cup Onions - chopped
- 1 (14.5 oz.) can diced Tomatoes
- 1 tsp. Bay Leaf (1 small leaf)
- Italian Seasoning, salt and pepper - both to taste
- 3/4 cup Green Beans - cut in 1-in pieces
- 3 oz. skinless chicken Breast - baked

Instructions:

- Cook the Green Beans to your liking - boil or steam Heat Olive Oil in medium size pan.
- Add onion and sauté' until tender.
- Add Tomatoes, Bay Leaf, Italian Seasoning, salt and pepper and chicken.
- Cover and let simmer 10 minutes.
- Drain excess liquid from beans and add to tomatoes and onion mixture.
- Cook 5 more minutes. Remove bay leaf before serving.

### Quick Delicious Salmon Patty - Serves 1

*Anti- Inflammatory Diet*
Ingredients:

- 3 oz. Bumble Bee Red Salmon
- 1 Egg White
- 1/3 cup old fashioned Rolled Oats
- 1/4 medium Onion - diced
- 1/2 clove Garlic - minced or to taste
- Salt and Pepper to taste
- 2/3 tsp. Olive Oil
- 4 leaves Romaine Lettuce
- 1 Tomato
- 1/2 Cucumber

Instructions:

- Flake Salmon in medium bowl.
- Add egg white, oats, onion, garlic, salt and pepper. Mix well with hands.
- Heat Olive Oil in pan on medium heat.
- Shape mixture into a patty.
- Cook 3-5 minutes on each side until golden brown.

Serve immediately on a lettuce, tomato, and cucumber bed.

# About The Author

Peyton Channing took an interest in finding out about the alternate methods that could be used to help alleviate the pain that comes with inflammation when his sister was diagnosed with rheumatoid arthritis. Though his sister was on prescribed medication, she would still have flare ups when the pain would be almost unbearable.

Peyton found out that there was an anti-inflammatory diet which could help to alleviate the pain. After his sister got the go ahead to try it from her rheumatologist, he saw that she was doing much better. This encouraged him to share his findings with others.

www.ingramcontent.com/pod-product-compliance
Ingram Content Group UK Ltd.
Pitfield, Milton Keynes, MK11 3LW, UK
UKHW022119230426
12048UKWH00010BA/611